Table of Conte

MW01598921

INTRODUCTION

I am sure that most people are familiar with the term detox cleansing diet and are aware of its benefits as well as some drawbacks in cases of some people. Also, in the detox cleansing diet one can find an overwhelming range of options which is why most people are actually confused whether to go for detoxification regimen or not. This diet basically helps to eliminate the buildup waste in your body along with making you lose a few pounds as well.

We have become exposed to an increasing number of chemicals in our food supply, the air we breathe, and through many common items, we use daily including cosmetics and household cleaner.

Among their potentially adverse effects, these chemicals can build up in our system and stall weight loss. While many factors often contribute, researchers find that environmental toxins play a role in being overweight or obese.

That's where a well-designed detoxification plan can help, like following the MaxLiving Detox System steps, which uses natural ingredients to support your body's detoxification process. Besides helping you eliminate the wrong foods that can contribute to weight gain, the right detox program can give your liver and overall health a helping hand eliminating those excess toxins.

"Detox diets range from total starvation fasts to juice fasts to food modification approaches and often involve the use of laxatives, diuretics, vitamins, minerals and/or 'cleansing foods,'"

So, if you are confused whether to go for a detox regime or not, this book will help you clear your doubts.

What Is Detox Cleansing Diet

Do you want to lose weight but don't know what the best diet program that is safe and effective? Have you heard about the detox cleansing diet that is commonly used by many? Cleansing is a good way of cleansing the body from the harmful toxins that can cause different illnesses.

The main goal of detox cleansing diet aside of losing weight is to cleanse the body's system from toxins, impurities and free radicals that have built-up over time. There are different detox diets and some of these diets are extreme than others. But most of these extreme diets are not mostly recommended by health experts because other people can't stick with this kind of diet.

Remember before starting a cleansing diet it is important to understand the effects of the food you are putting into your body. Many foods today that are commonly thought to be part of a good balanced diet can actually harm the body. During the cleansing period, you need to avoid preserved foods, meat, dairy products, sweet foods, hydrogenated fats, oily foods and drugs.

In this period, you should only consume whole grains, vegetables, fruits, soy, wheat, beans, fish and herbs. The more natural the diet is the better it is good for the body. If possible, consume only vegetables because it is healthiest for your body and it is rich in fibre that helps speed up metabolism. It is also important that you need to have a good metabolic rate to burn also the unwanted fats in the body.

Another easy way to cleanse the body is by drinking water at least a gallon of water a day. You can also drink natural herbal teas, natural lemon juice, and other fresh juices and eliminate carbonated sodas, diet sodas and coffee that contain caffeine. This is a good way of flushing out the toxins and maintaining the bowel movement.

Aside from the foods that you must eat, exercising regularly is also an excellent way to help the body rid itself of toxins through perspiration. So it is advice that you must include exercising daily in your regimen. It will not only cleanse your system but will also make you lose weight.

It is believed that the length of time a cleansing diet is maintained is based on the person's need. A detox cleansing diet is unlike other usual diets because it can be maintained indefinitely and become a life style choice for some people who will get used to it. It can also be used periodically to help give your body a boost when you feel it is needed to make you feel healthy all the time.

Besides the benefits mentioned above about the diet, many people prefer it because it is their way of preventing certain illnesses and conditions like liver malfunction, kidney problems, hormonal imbalance, nutritional deficiencies etc. So with the help of a detox diet it will improve your energy, complexion, bowel movement, metabolism and digestion. So what more can you ask for in this diet, for it will improve wellness and of course your well being.

Background

The idea of detoxing the body dates back thousands of years. In fact, several sources say that the process of detoxification can be traced back to ancient Egyptian and biblical times. Native Americans used ritual cleansing and purification to remove toxins. And in the early 20th-century, bloodletting, enemas, and fasting were detox methods used by the legitimate medical community.

In short, the idea of getting rid of body toxins to boost health and wellness is a concept that has been—and continues to be—an appealing one. Unfortunately, however, the concept is not backed by strong scientific evidence, at least not as a general health or wellness concept.1

In clinical settings, the term "detox" is used to refer to a medical process that rids the body of alcohol, drugs, or poisons. Detox treatments are provided in a hospital or clinic setting under the care of a licensed professional and may involve the use of medications and other therapies.

But detox diets are a different concept. Many of these programs claim to rid the body of toxins that we are exposed to in the process of normal activities. Some research suggests that many of the chemicals we ingest daily through food, water, and air can become deposited in fat cells in our bodies.2

Those who promote and sell some detox programs claim that by ridding the body of this waste, you might enjoy health benefits including a boost of energy,

11

clearer skin, weight loss, and other advantages. The problem is that aren't high-quality, independent, clinical studies to support these claims.

Authors of a critical review investigated the body's response to common toxins called persistent organic pollutants (POPs). The authors concluded that there was not enough scientific evidence to support the idea that POPs provide any harm to the body or that there is a need to eliminate them.2

In fact, your body already has systems in place to rid itself of harmful toxins. We absorb toxins through our skin, in the air that we breathe, and in the food that we eat. But our body's organs—primarily the liver, kidneys, colon, and lungs have systems in place to flush out these contaminants naturally.

In short, your body is always in a state of detoxification. Each of these organs has a different role.

• The liver plays a key role by filtering the blood and removing harmful substances that occur as a result of normal body functions (like digestion) or external toxins like drugs, alcohol, or chemicals.

• The kidneys also help filter the blood and remove toxins in the form of urine.

• After nutrients are removed from food in the small intestine, the colon (or large intestine) filters the remaining waste, including toxins, to be excreted.

• Cilia in the lungs trap toxins that enter the body in the air that you breathe. These contaminants are then expelled by coughing or through other natural body processes.

So while it is true that our bodies are exposed to pollutants, there is scant evidence that our body needs help in removing them. In fact, eating a nutritious diet to support healthy cells and organs may be the smartest way to boost detoxification.

But not all detox diets make claims about pollutants. Some detox plans are designed simply to "retrain" your tastebuds so that you crave healthier foods, or reduce your intake of less nutritious foods in an effort to boost wellness. Less restrictive detox diet plans like these may provide benefits if they are used as a springboard to a longer term plan for healthy eating.

There are many different types of detox diets. Some are short-term, lasting just a few days while others last several weeks. The foods or beverages on each detox program can vary substantially as well.

Unfortunately, there is no clear consensus in the health community about which foods are most effective when the goal is to detoxify the body.

Authors of a 2015 study published in the Journal of Nutrition and Metabolism were able to identify certain foods including garlic, grapefruit, rosemary, and different types of tea that may be more effective for detoxification. But those researchers also suggested consumers should get a meal plan from a trained clinician noting that "there remain many unresolved issues regarding knowing how and what foods modulate detoxification pathways."3

While there are no clear guidelines regarding a specific detox food list, there are a few trends among the most popular programs. Almost all detox diets eliminate processed foods such as lunchmeat, refined bread or pasta, and foods that contain added sugar or excess sodium. Many detox programs limit your food intake to fruits, vegetables, and lean meats. The most restrictive plans include only juice drinks and no solid foods.

The healthiest detox programs will allow you to eat from all of the food groups identified in the nutritional guidelines developed by the US Department of Agriculture (USDA) and Health and Human Services

(HHS), including vegetables, fruit, grains, fat-free or low-fat dairy, protein foods, and healthy oils. Detox programs that include these food groups are not common.

What Are Toxins?

The word "toxin" is often used to refer to chemical substances or pollutants including:

• Pesticides

• Antibiotics or hormones in food

• Chemicals from food packaging

• Household cleaners

• Detergents

- Food additives

- Heavy metals

- Air pollution

- Drugs

- Cigarette smoke

Why A Detox Cleansing Diet is the Best Diet For You

There are many kinds of diet out there but most people prefer the detox cleansing diet. But why do most people prefer this kind of diet among the different diets out there? What are the benefits that we can get from this kind of diet?

Yes it's true that there are many kinds of diet programs out there but still the detox diet is the most preferred diet by most people and even celebrities. What I know about this diet is that it cleanses our body to prevent the body from certain ailments. Cleansing is a good way of eliminating the body from toxins and wastes that was accumulated from foods and even on the environment that we are living.

This is the main goal of this diet, to cleanse the body and make it free from toxins. These toxins are the reason why people get sick and suffer from different illnesses such as heart attack, stroke, hypertension, stomach problems and diabetes. So in order to prevent people from these illnesses, they should start this kind of diet now.

In a detox diet, this is the diet where you have to consume lots of fruits and vegetables and in the same time drinking lots of water a day. These foods are rich in nutrients and fibre that is a good aid in cleansing. Water also is a good solvent that helps in digestion and regulating bowel movement.

While in the process of the diet, you should never eat foods such as sweet and fatty foods, preserved foods, junk foods, dairy products, salty foods and oily foods. These foods are full of toxins that clog the pathways of the organs that make the organs not to function well. This is the reason why some people feel tired, lethargy, sluggish, dull and sick.

So to prevent this from happening, you must go on this kind of diet. It not only helps you lose weight, it also helps you get rid of toxins that could cause illnesses. But remember, before going on diet like this, you need to consult your doctor first. There are some circumstances that there are people who are not a good candidate for this kind of diet so for your safety seek your doctor first.

The length of detoxification depends on the person's needs. If he had felt that he had consume lots of toxins because he had live an unhealthy lifestyle then the process of detoxification will really take long. What's also good about this detox cleansing diet is that it can be maintained indefinitely as long as your body can handle it.

Now you know why the detox cleansing diet is the best among the other diets out there. It not only makes you lose weight but is also helps in cleansing the body for a healthier you. If you want to experience the lightness in your body then try it now and live a healthy life from now on.

The Benefits Of A Detox Cleanse Diet

Many so-called detox cleanse diets have things like amphetamines and caffeine incorporated in their detox cleanse formula, which is not a true cleanse but more of a stimulant to temporarily control your appetite, and as soon as you finish the "cleansing" process, you will ultimately end up being hungrier and gaining back all the weight, if not more.

When deciding on a detox cleanse diet, you should keep this checklist in mind:

* Does the diet truly "cleanse" my body?

* Will the diet bring my pH back into balance causing my metabolism to speed up?

* Does the cleanse deprive my body of the much-needed electrolytes such as salt and potassium, causing me to lose only water, not fat?

* What organs of the body is the diet actually cleansing?

* Are the products all natural or dangerous chemicals?

* What am I cleansing my body from?

* Can I cleanse my body from bad carbs?

These are just a few questions you may want to ask of yourself and find out the answer before beginning any form of a body cleansing diet.

There are actually many different forms of cleansing that can take place in the body through very natural means. For instance, cleansing the liver can be easily done with grapefruit and olive oil. Apple cider vinegar cleanses the blood, brings your pH levels into balance, ultimately causing your metabolism to speed up.

Also, did you know that when you start any type of low carb diet, you're actually entering into a category of cleansing, detoxifying your body from the harmful, diabetes-producing effects of harmful carbs, helping you to lose weight as well as protect yourself from the diabetes?

So, remember, before starting any type of detox cleanse diet, make sure it's natural and above all safe.

2014 was the year of the cleanse diet. Celebrities swear by them and more and more people have been getting in on the action, whether it's to detox diet, brighten skin, lose weight, or get a fresh start. And nowhere is that more evident than in Yahoo's Year in Review, where different health cleanses consistently topped the site's most popular stories lists. Here, the year's top 10 most popular cleanses:

1. **A Colon Cleanse.** Our colons have the important, albeit kind of icky, job of taking digested food from our stomachs, pulling the nutrients out, and excreting waste. While for most of us, our colons perform their duties just fine, every once in a while you might feel like giving a helping hand, er, enema. Colon cleanses come

25

in many different types, methods, and prices, but the main idea is to use water, fiber, and/or supplements to flush all the gunk out of your intestines so you can start fresh.

2. **A Liver Cleanse.** Just like our colons, our livers play an important role in ridding our bodies of unwanted toxins. The three-pound organ sits just under your ribs and is responsible for cleaning your blood. Some people believe that eating certain foods or taking certain supplements can help your liver perform better-or help it when it's overwhelmed by too many trips through the drive-thru. However, experts caution that most "liver detox" products don't work as advertised. Some can actually cause harm to your liver as the organ is responsible for metabolizing any drugs, medications, or

herbals supplements. In fact, diet supplements are the number two cause for hospitalizations for liver damage- and the Food and Drug Administration (FDA) has issued a warning against these types of detoxes.

3. The Master Cleanse. While the Master Cleanse has been around for decades, it was Beyonce who made it mainstream. She used the diet to drop some serious weight for her role in Dreamgirls. To do it, you drink a concoction of lemon water, maple syrup, and cayenne pepper, along with an herbal detox tea, daily for at least 10 days-and nothing else. While it may work in the short term, experts say it isn't safe long-term. And even Miss B said it was "awful" and made her "cranky."

4. The 10-Day Green Smoothie Cleanse. Pictures of green smoothies have probably been all over your

Facebook feed for months as this popular cleanse has spread through social media. Participants say they drop up to 15 pounds by drinking only smoothies made of blended fruits and veggies for 10 days, as outlined by J.J. Smith's popular book. While the diet is high in vitamins, minerals, and fiber, it lacks other important nutrients, like protein

5. A Juice Cleanse. Juicing has long been used as a way to get lots of vitamins and minerals from fruits and vegetables without having to, well, eat all those fruits and vegetables. So juice cleanses, of which there are many different types, take advantage of this vitamin mega-dose by having people replace all (or part) of their solid food with specially formulated juices. While the cleanses can be a great way to get your daily produce in, experts warn that many juices are high in sugar and lack the fiber that whole fruit has

6. Detox Cleanse. Detoxing-or removing unhealthy toxins from the body-is one of the main reasons people give for wanting to do a cleanse. Toxic overload can make you feel sluggish, lead to acne, and can cause allergic reactions-among a host of other ills. But most experts warn against pill- or drink-based detox cleanses. The body's own mechanisms for cleansing using the liver, kidneys, and colon are sufficient to rid your body of most toxins, they say. Thankfully, there are lots of healthy changes you can make to support your body while it does all the tough detox work

7. Slendera Garcinia and Natural Cleanse. Garcinia Cambogia is a supplement made from the tropical fruit that bears its name (also known as tamarind). It's high in fiber and boosts serotonin levels in your brain, possibly helping you feel full faster and longer. Slendera is one brand name of a garcinia cambogia supplement that is often combined with a larger cleansing plan involving "natural" laxatives and diuretics. Most experts advise steering clear of laxatives and diuretics, natural or otherwise, unless your doctor advises you to take them for a specific reason. Long-term use can be very harmful to your body. However, garcinia cambogia extracts may offer a small boost for dieters.

8. Dherbs Full Body Cleanse. Dherbs is a company that makes a line of proprietary supplements that claim to cure a range of illnesses and health problems. The Full Body Cleanse is a system of pills or liquid supplements you take on a daily basis for 20 days in addition to following a suggested raw-food diet. Proponents say they have lost nearly a pound a day and feel more energized. However, because of the limited information available on the company's site, not much is known about what exactly is in the supplements-or how they work. Still interested? You should note they're pretty pricey and the company has a no-refund policy after the bottle is opened.

9. Blueprint Cleanse. A celebrity favorite and "2012 diet of the year," the Blueprint Cleanse is a pre-packaged juice cleanse in which you are sent six bottles of vegan juices made from fruits, vegetables, and spices, customized to your health goals. You drink the juices-and nothing else-for periods ranging from three days to two weeks. The company says their plans range from 860 to 1,040 calories per day. While this is not specifically billed as a weight-loss cleanse, you probably will drop some pounds.

10. Isagenix Cleanse for Life. Isagenix is a multi-level marketing company that specializes in wellness supplements, liquids and powders, along with some snack and meal-replacement products. The Cleanse for Life is a specific supplement that comes in either powder or liquid form which the company recommends be used as part of one of their larger cleansing systems. Proponents say it helps drop weight, increase energy and cure many ailments.

Are cleansing diets new?

Cleansing diets aren't new. "They've been around for years and years," Mangieri says. But they seem to get a lot of press from magazines and talk show hosts. And celebrities make cleanse diets popular every time they claim to lose significant weight on them.

"The terms 'detox' and 'cleanse' have become almost interchangeable and are thrown around almost as much as the words 'calorie' and 'carbohydrate' these days," says Keri Glassman, RD, CDN, founder and president of A Nutritious Life, a nutrition practice based in New York City.

Proponents of cleansing diets believe it's important to rid your body of toxins that you get -- like it or not --

from food, water and the environment. "The mistake most people make is equating detoxes and cleanses with weight loss," Glassman says. They are not the same.

So if you're considering a cleanse diet as a way to lose weight, you could be outsmarting yourself. "Cleanse diets can set you up for failure by slowing your metabolism and making you crave everything you just gave up," Glassman says. Cleanse diets don't help you or your body develop healthy eating habits. And what's worse, they could deprive your body of essential nutrients, Mangieri agrees.

Can your body cleanse itself?

Glassman says it's not necessary to go on a special diet to "clean" your digestive system. "Our bodies are natural systems built to detox all the time," she says. "Our liver, skin, urinary system, and gastrointestinal tract are constantly helping to cleanse our bodies through sweat, urine and feces."

Eating a diet high in fiber, drinking lots of water, and avoiding packaged and processed foods are major ways to keep your body working optimally. "Such a diet will ensure that your body is cleansing as naturally as it can," Glassman says.

What is a modified cleansing diet?

Glassman never recommends that anyone go on an extreme (all liquid) cleanse diet, especially not for an extended period of time. However, she says a modified version may help you reboot your system, especially if you overindulged on vacation or have gotten into a fast-food rut.

In her book, The New You and Improved Diet, Glassman recommends a four-day regimen that some people may find helpful. It consists of eight foods:

• artichokes,

• avocados,

• eggs,

• granny smith apples,

• lentils,

• olive oil,

• salmon, and

• spinach.

"I chose these foods because as a group they offer healthy fat, protein, fiber, and water volume. Plus they're loaded with antioxidants," she says.

Glassman says eating only these foods for three or four days will help you feel better. That timeframe also can be enough to "set up new healthy behaviors," she says.

Making healthy food choices will help you feel better. "Feeling physically and mentally better will help motivate you to stick with [it] for three to four days," Glassman says. "It also may motivate you to continue to incorporate the healthy habits you learn into your daily life.

Detox Cleansing Diet - How to Lose Weight & Gain Energy!

The Master cleansing diet is the most well known of the detox cleaning diets and works wonders. This is the one that Hollywood tried to keep secrets, and even celebrities like Beyonce have used it to lose weight and become healthier. It is time you learned about all the benefits of a detox cleansing diet.

We are going to discuss a few of the key benefits and they are all important to your overall health. These benefits combined can help you change your entire physical body. Here are few of the top benefits of a cleansing diet for you to mull over.

The first benefit you will notice will be more stamina and energy. This one is a big deal and you will notice it pretty quickly after you complete your detox. You will be cleaning your body of all the sludge in it so you will feel less weighed down and more energetic. Plus the energy you are helping to create will also help you heal better.

Did you know that this increase in energy will also give you a lot more time each week? What would you do with an extra hour each day? More time comes from the body being able to get by with less sleep and with more energy you will be able to complete tasks faster than normal.

You will also experience a renewal in your health. This is like the way we deal with the common cold. When we get sick it is all fluids and no solids. This allows our body to use our digestive energy to help fight off the cold. It is similar with a detox, but you will be healing areas that you didn't even know needed to be healed.

The renewal you will experience will change your overall health by leaps and bounds. This is something that is known to be used for healing with athletes and others as well. It will allow you to recover from chronic soreness much faster as well.

The third benefit is very important. You will increase your motivation, focus and self discipline. Doing a detox cleansing is not exactly easy and many will fail. However, when you complete your cleansing you will have gained focus, self discipline, and it will be a way to test your motivation.

Of course, the last benefit is the Weight Loss you will experience from the detox cleansing diet. Most people will lose between 5 and 7 pounds, but there have been some that lose as much as 20 pounds. This is quite a bit to cut over a 10 day period. This happens because you will be forcing toxins out of your body while allowing your body to work off the existing fat for a short period of time.

How to Prepare for a Detox Cleanse

Do you know that your body needs to be cleansed every once in a while? This is because it accumulates a lot of toxins; harmful substances that weaken the immune system. It may be the reason why more often than not, you feel so consumed after a day's work. When these contaminants are not removed from your body, chances are that you will be more prone to acquiring diseases like fever, colds and other bacterial infections. Thankfully, there are is a simple way to renew your body, and that is through the detox cleanse.

Detoxification is important in order to return your body to its natural condition. It can help restore the bodily processes in order to have a sound physiology and psyche. You will be able to relieve stress and, at the same time, bring back lost energy and enthusiasm. All of these can be done with the right cleansing diet.

You may think that cleansing can be done simply by lessening your food consumption or by incorporating lots of fruits and vegetables in your diet. While this could work, it may not be enough. The proper detox cleanse has a more detailed action plan that you should follow. To start, you must first assess your stress level. This will give you a fairly good idea as to how much toxins are in your body. The higher the stress level, the longer you need to engage in a cleansing diet.

It is also better to consult a nutritionist or a dietician before pushing through with the diet. Let them check on your health just to make sure that the detox cleanse will be effective for you. The nutritionist can even help set up a proper program that you can follow to make sure that you still acquire your daily nutritional needs while doing the detoxification process.

Lastly, determine what kind of cleansing diet you wish to follow. There are many types of diets that are available and it is important that you do some research first. Pick a diet that you can easily commit to and make sure that it will not interfere with your daily routine.

What To Look Out For When On The Master Cleanse Diet

People are facing various health issues due to increasing body weight and as a result they are looking for many methods to reduce the body weight. It mainly includes various diet methods for slimming down but the result is always turning to be negative. Also some of them are not in a position to carry out some of the dieting methods due to unavailability of certain dieting ingredients mentioned in the diet plan. The Master cleanse diet has turned out to be the most prominent one which every one prefer these days. It is really effective but still there are certain difficulties faced by some and some are actually not aware about the side effects before starting the dieting process.

The master cleanse diet actually came into being long back in the year 1941 and was invented by Stanley Burroughs. This diet was developed to get rid of all the unwanted toxic materials that are getting deposited in the body with the passage of time. These materials are deposited in the body through the means of consumption of various food items like caffeine and other junk food that are made out of various chemical substances. It is also widely spoken that the diet process can help in cleaning the body along with the measures of preventive for some diseases like cancer and ulcers that are caused by the presence of toxins inside the human body.

This diet is initially designed for a time period of 10 days and the diet is moving with the help of only liquid food items made from fresh vegetables and fruits. You are not supposed to take any other food items during this period other than liquid food. Also you are not supposed to take water without mixing with fresh juice. You should completely say no to the beverages, coffee, tea and so on. Some people would like to extend the diet days to 30 or 90 in order to reduce the required amount of body weight.

You should try very well to understand the concept about the master cleanse diet before actually starting the procedure. This diet plan is designed only for the removing the toxic particles from the body and not for the purpose of reducing body weight. Therefore you are advised to carry on with the diet only for the prescribed number of days rather than increasing the time period. There are many toxic particles in the body and these mainly include the presence of pesticides, insecticides, heavy metals, and so on and such a cleansing process is very essential for removing the particles from the body rather than leading to various infections. You can some times experience certain side effects like vomiting, stomach pain, and headache and so on while undergoing the cleansing process.

It is very clear that when you start having your normal food items naturally your body weight will add leading to the usual stage. The slim figure will last only for short time frame and this is mainly due to the lower metabolic rate in you while carrying on with the dieting process. It is strongly advised to avoid the practice of master cleanse diet mainly for the purpose of body weight reduction.

How to Choose an Effective Detox Cleanse Product

Detox cleanse is now becoming more popular and it is usually the process recommended by practitioners of natural health. The main reason for this can be the fact that around half of the immune system lies in an area that is around the digestive system. This means that the body won't be able to absorb enough nutrients unless the colon is cleaned and the toxins that have accumulated in it have been eliminated. If the toxins that accumulate in the colon through the food we eat are left alone, they could become a hindrance to proper digestion and can cause other health disorders such as bloating, headaches, bad breath, constipation, infections, fatigue allergies and obesity.

Studies have shown that effective cleansing of the colon can be achieved by dieting, fasting, taking a lot of water and using detox cleanse products. There are a lot of such products on the market though and choosing the most effective one for you can be confusing. Hence, you must have a list of considerations when doing your shopping.

One of these is the right ingredients. You have to make sure that the product you will buy will be effective and only high quality ingredients are used. You should also look at the all the feedback given by costumers about the product. If there are negative feedback given to a product by various costumers, stay away from it.

Many colon cleansing products have offers that will let you sample them at minimum costs. This is a good indication that the product can work as intended since the manufacturer is willing to back it up with a guarantee.

Remember that it is easy to make claims about the effectiveness of a product so what you should be looking for are results. The company should also be able to assume the risk of having its costumers try their detox cleanse products for free so that they can decide for themselves.

Never Do a Liver Cleansing Diet That Ignores the Lymph! A Good Body Detox Diet Includes Lymphatics!

A liver cleansing diet is a little misleading because it doesn't only help your liver but also benefits the rest of your body. So a liver cleansing diet is really a liver cleanser for your whole body. For example, did you know that your liver directly affects the lymph? Important? You bet.

51

Lymph is the interstitial fluid found between cells of the human body. It enters the lymph vessels by filtering through pores in the walls of capillaries, then travels to at least one lymph node before emptying into the right or the left subclavian vein, where it mixes back with blood.

Huh?

Without good lymph movement, toxins and waste build up in the body, causing enlarged lymph nodes, tiredness, skin problems, sinus problems, headaches and a weakened immune system. If you're serious about doing a whole body detox then looking after your lymph is just part of it. And a liver cleansing diet is a great liver cleanser for a healthy detox.

Best Ways for Lymph Circulation

1. One of the best exercises for lymph circulation is gentle bouncing on a rebounder. These days rebounders only cost between $30-$60. The best part; they can be packed under your bed, in a closet or behind a door. The important part is to use it!

2. A big problem causing sluggish lymph is in activity - so sitting for long periods does you no favors. And a huge reminder for those of us behind a computer a lot of the time. If you get lost in your work and forget to move around use a digital timer and set it for every hour - if not less - to get up, walk around and grab a glass of purified water or a freshly squeezed juice.

3. Dry brushing is a great self-massage to wake up your arms, chest, face, and neck. It's an easy, inexpensive

way to get your lymph active. Start by brushing the soles of your feet, briskly in a circular motion. Using short, upward strokes, moving from your feet and up your legs, over your stomach to your breasts and over your buttocks to your waist. Repeat the circular motion on the palms of your hands and use short, upward strokes up your arms. Brush down your neck to your shoulders and inwards across your breasts towards your heart. With time your skin will improve and you can stroke harder.

These three simple activities will benefit your lymph and you enormously, dramatically increasing the elimination of fats and toxins out of your system and decreasing belly-fattening levels of cortisol and lowering stress. Great trade off if you ask me.

These three simple steps will help your lymph to saturate your body with enzymes, antioxidants and phytonutrients to support, detoxify and eliminate deposits of lymphatic waste - and reduce cellulite. The benefits just keep on coming.

Don't do these simple activities and you leave out one of the most important steps of any natural detoxification program. In fact, most body detox diets forget to include lymph circulation when detoxing when now we have a new breed of toxins to add to the list.

1. Pesticides and preservatives create estrogen imitators,

2. Electromagnetic fields (EMFs) from cell phones and other Wi-Fi sources,

3. Plastics and perchlorate (from rocket fuel), antibiotics and other drugs in our water supplies.

In today's toxic world, ignoring the liver and lymph can make you very sick. In fact, you'd be stupid not to use a healthy detox that includes them.

Your body needs serious heavy-duty nutritional support to break down toxins:

1. Eat liver friendly vegetables such as broccoli, cabbage, cauliflower - speeding the elimination of fat-storing toxins.

2. Add eggs preferably organic eggs to your diet to get the sulfur and lecithin you need to support the liver's detox pathways.

There are even more benefits for having a healthy lymphatic system. Apart from glowing, smooth skin and a toned body, nutrients become more available to your body's cells. Sugar cravings cease. Swelling and bloating disappear.

So start your liver cleansing diet with your lymphatic system in mind - never sit in one place for too long, dry brush your skin at least once a week and look at some exercise like rebounding that gets the blood flowing quickly. Remember the best liver cleansing diet is whole body cleanse using natural detoxification at its core to give you a healthy detox.

These liver cleansing diets don't cost a lot of money - but they do need action.

Pros and Cons of a Detox Cleanse Diet

Many consumers choose to go on detox diet programs because they provide quick weight loss. While you are not likely to lose fat on a short-term program, you are likely to lose some water weight, especially on a low-carb detox. Your clothes might fit better and you might feel lighter.

Another benefit of these plans is that they are short-lived. A three-day program is much more palatable for some and may provide a stepping stone to healthier habits.

If the thought of a permanent diet overhaul seems overwhelming, a short detox may provide you with an opportunity to improve your nutritional intake to boost wellness. If you like the way it feels, you may feel motivated to make changes that stick.

The problem, however, is that without a plan to transition to a long-term program for healthy eating, any benefits that you gain on a detox diet are likely to disappear when you return to your typical eating pattern.

In fact, authors of one study published in Current Gastroenterology Reports compared different diets, including detox diets. They concluded that "juicing and detoxification diets tend to work because they lead to extremely low caloric intake for short periods of time, however, they tend to lead to weight gain once a normal diet is resumed."4

And if the detox diet that you choose is very low in calories, you may even gain weight from unhealthy binging after the detox is complete. Studies have shown that when a diet is very restrictive, you put yourself at higher risk for binge eating and weight gain. 5

Herbal Detox Cleanse

There's no doubt that over the past 15 years or so, cleansing and detox have become increasingly popular. A practice that was once limited to "health nuts" and people with serious diseases is now commonplace. But what is the best way to cleanse?

The major detox methods include:

• Fasting

• Cleansing by changing your diet

• Colonics

• Drinking special teas

• And Herbal Detox

Most alternative health practitioners consider the herbal detox cleanse to be the most effective strategy for long term detox. There are 3 main reasons for this.

First, cleansing with herbs supports all three of the major detox organs simultaneously. In a high quality cleansing program you'll find specific herbs to address the colon, the liver and the kidneys. Other approaches to detox simply can't compete on that level. Colon hydrotherapy only works with the colon. Fasting, when done over a long period, can actually stress the liver rather than support it. Drinking special teas have some effect but require a long period to really work.

The second reason that an herbal detox cleanse is considered to be so effective is that the best programs require that you make positive changes to your diet while your taking the herbal formulas. Cleansing with herbs is not a "take an aspirin and call me tomorrow" approach. It works over time and requires that you also make healthy changes in your eating habits. That means eliminating foods that slow digestion like meats, dairy products and processed foods while including plenty of fresh fruits and vegetables.

The third aspect of a quality herbal detox cleanse that makes it shine as an approach to detox is that it easier to complete than other approaches. Unlike colon hydrotherapy, it involves absolutely no invasive procedures nor the risks associated with them. Unlike fasting you still get to eat while on an herbal cleansing program. And an herbal detox cleanse can work much faster than a detox regime based only on changing your diet.

If you're ready to make those positive, life affirming changes in your life that you've longed for, consider herbal detox as a way to get to your goals. A quality program will leave you feeling lighter, healthier and most likely a lot happier than when you started.

How do you know if you need to detoxify?

Bennett suggests that everyone should detox at least once a year. However, Bennett cautions against detoxing for nursing mothers, children, and patients with chronic degenerative diseases, cancer or tuberculosis. Consult your healthcare practitioner if you have questions about whether detoxing is right for you.

Today, with more toxins in the environment than ever, "it's critical to detox," says Linda Page, N.D., Ph.D., the author of Detoxification: Programs to Cleanse, Purify and Renew. Page recommends detoxing for symptoms such as:

• Unexplained fatigue

• Sluggish elimination

• Irritated skin

• Allergies

• Low-grade infection

• Puffy eyes or bags under the eyes

• Bloating

• Menstrual problems

• Mental confusion

How do you start a detox?

First, lighten up your toxin load. Eliminate alcohol, coffee, cigarettes, refined sugars, and saturated fats, all of which act as toxins in the body and are obstacles to your healing process. Also, minimize use of chemical-based household cleaners and personal health care products (cleansers, shampoos, deodorants, and toothpastes), and substitute natural alternatives.

Another hindrance to good health is stress, which triggers your body to release stress hormones into your system. While these hormones can provide the "adrenaline rush" to win a race or meet a deadline, in large amounts they create toxins and slow down detoxification enzymes in the liver. Yoga, Qigong and meditation are simple and effective ways to relieve stress by resetting your physical and mental reactions to the inevitable stress life will bring. Gaiam carries yoga mats, props and accessories for beginner yogis to advanced practitioners and a meditation seating to help you relieve stress.

Which detox program is right for you?

There are many detoxification programs and detox recipes, depending on your individual needs. Many programs follow a seven-day schedule because, as Bennett explains, "it takes the body time to clean the blood." His program involves fasting on liquids for two days, followed by a carefully planned five-day detox diet to allow the digestive system to rest. Page recommends a three- to seven-day juice fast (drinking only fresh fruit and vegetable juices and water) as an effective way to release toxins.

Here are our five favorite detox diets:

1. Simple Fruit and Veggie Detox

2. Smoothie Cleanse

3. Juice Cleanse

4. Sugar Detox

5. Hypoallergenic Detox

Top 10 ways to help your body detoxify

After a detoxification program, you can cleanse your body daily with these diet supplements and lifestyle practices:

1. Eat plenty of fiber, including brown rice and organically grown fresh fruits and vegetables. Beets, radishes, artichokes, cabbage, broccoli, spirulina, chlorella, and seaweed are excellent detoxifying foods.

2. Cleanse and protect the liver by taking herbs such as dandelion root, burdock, and milk thistle, and drinking green tea.

3. Take vitamin C, which helps the body produce glutathione, a liver compound that drives away toxins.

4. Drink at least two quarts of water a day, made easy by bringing our 32 oz. Stainless Steel Wide Mouth Water Bottle with you everywhere you go!

5. Breathe deeply to allow oxygen to circulate more completely through your system.

6. Transform stress by emphasizing positive emotions.

7. Practice hydrotherapy by taking a very hot shower for five minutes, allowing the water to run on your back.

Follow with cold water for 30 seconds. Do this three times, and then get into bed for 30 minutes.

8. Sweat in a sauna so your body can eliminate waste through perspiration.

9. Dry-brush your skin or try detox foot spas/foot baths to remove toxins through your pores. Special brushes are available at natural products stores.

10. What's the most important way to detoxify? "Exercise," says Bennett. "Yoga or jump-roping are good. One hour every day." Also try Qigong, a martial arts based exercise system that includes exercises specifically for detoxifying or cleansing, as well as many other exercises with specific health benefits.

The 7-Day Detox Diet Plan: Time to Get Healthy & Active

Smooth digestion and absorption of nutrients along with your liver's efficient processing of toxins are absolutely critical for great health. That's why a cleanse program can be a powerful tool to rejuvenate your body and skin from the inside out.

The key to comfortable cleanse is to ease yourself into the program, so that your body doesn't go into a shock. Five days before you begin your detox diet plan, progressively eliminate alcohol, coffee, cigarettes, refined sugars, saturated fats and all processed foods. These can add as toxins in your body.

Increase fiber intake to help keep your colon clean. Along with the fiber from fruits and vegetables, include two tablespoon of chia seeds in a glass of water to eliminate toxins from your body. Don't forget to drink lots of filtered water- at least eight glasses per day.

Another deterrent to good health is stress, as it triggers your body to release stress hormones. It's a good idea to cleanse stressful life situations along with your body. Keep a diary and take a note not only of what you eat and drink but also your emotions.

I hope you are sufficiently motivated, now let's get started with the specifics of your personal detox diet plan.

DAY 1

Start the morning with half a lemon squeezed into warm water or cleansing herb tea. Follow with a brisk walk, bike ride, yoga or swimming.

BREAKFAST: Fresh vegetables juice (choose from the list below)

Carrots, Beetroot, Celery, Mint, Coriander, Parsley, Wheatgrass, Spinach, Kale

Add a tablespoon of chia seeds to your juice, for that extra fiber and power boost. (I don't recommend juicing fruits as that will shoot up your sugar levels and we don't want that happening).

LUNCH: Raw or lightly steamed vegetables with a variety of seasonal preferably organic vegetables .

You can choose from the following:

Mushrooms, Spinach, Mustard leaves, Fenugreek leaves, Beetroot, Broccoli, Cabbage, Capsicums, Pumpkins, Carrots, Onions, Garlic, Ginger

DINNER: Vegetable stew

In a large saucepan, saute onions and garlic. Then add your favourite veggies, saute for another 2 minutes. Add 2 cups of filtered water and sea salt. Slow cook till the veggies are done. You could blend the ingredients for a thick broth or eat it as is with chunks of veggies.

SNACKS: Drink as much water, unsweetened herbal tea as you wish during the day. Aim for at least 8 glass of

water within the day. Make a trail mix of nuts and seeds like walnuts, almonds, pumpkin seeds, sunflower seeds, melon seeds, chia seeds and flax seeds. Eat low GI fruits like guava, pear, apple, orange, strawberries, peach, plums and apricots.

DAY 2

Start the morning with half a lemon squeezed into warm water or cleansing herb tea. Follow with a brisk walk, bike ride, yoga or swimming

BREAKFAST: Fresh vegetable juice with 1 table spoon of chia seeds blended in. Choose from the list of juicing vegetables provided earlier.

LUNCH: Lightly cooked vegetables with quinoa and baby spinach salad.

DINNER: Vegetable stew with stir-fried red and yellow capsicums and broccoli, tossed with extra virgin olive oil, lemon juice and garlic.

SNACKS: Drink as much water, unsweetened herbal tea as you wish during the day. Aim for at least 8 glass of water within the day. Make a trail mix of nuts and seeds like walnuts, almonds, pumpkin seeds, sunflower seeds, melon seeds, chia seeds and flax seeds. Eat low GI fruits like guava, pear, apple, orange, strawberries, peach, plums and apricots.

DAY 3

Start the morning with half a lemon squeezed into warm water or cleansing herb tea. Follow with a brisk walk, bike ride, yoga or swimming.

BREAKFAST: 3/4 of cup of natural yoghurt with sliced fresh fruits, sprinkle with chia seeds, sliced almonds and walnuts and drizzle with a little raw honey if desired. You can follow this with green tea or herb tea.

LUNCH: Lentil and Vegetable Stew

Saute 1/2 cup of yellow moong dal, 1 cup of your favourite veggies, small pieces of ginger and two cloves of garlic in some extra virgin olive oil. Add 2 cups of water and salt to taste. Slow cook till the dal and veggies are done, garnish with coriander or parsley.

DINNER: Raw Papaya and Carrot Salad

Toss 2 cups of lettuce, 1 grated carrot and 1/2 raw papaya together. Mix 1 tablespoon of balsamic vinegar and 1 tablespoon of extra virgin olive oil, fresh lemon juice and drizzle over the top.

SNACKS: Drink as much water, unsweetened herbal tea as you wish during the day. Aim for at least 8 glass of water within the day. Make a trail mix of nuts and seeds like walnuts, almonds, pumpkin seeds, sunflower seeds, melon seeds, chia seeds and flax seeds. Eat low GI fruits like guava, pear, apple, orange, strawberries, peach, plums and apricots.

Start the morning with half a lemon squeezed into warm water or cleansing herb tea. Follow with a brisk walk, bike ride, yoga or swimming

BREAKFAST: Coconut Banana Power Smoothie

100 grams of natural yoghurt or organic coconut milk, 1 tablespoon of cold pressed coconut oil, and 1 or 1/2 banana, 1 tablespoon of chia seeds. Blend the ingredients in a high speed blender.

LUNCH: 1 bowl of vegetable stew with a cup of quinoa or amaranth.

DINNER: Lentil and vegetable Stew.

SNACKS: Drink as much water, unsweetened herbal tea as you wish during the day. Aim for at least 8 glass of

water within the day. Make a trail mix of nuts and seeds like walnuts, almonds, pumpkin seeds, sunflower seeds, melon seeds, chia seeds and flax seeds. Eat low GI fruits like guava, pear, apple, orange, strawberries, peach, plums and apricots.

DAY 5

Start the morning with half a lemon squeezed into warm water or cleansing herb tea. Follow with a brisk walk, bike ride, yoga or swimming

BREAKFAST: Fresh vegetable juice with 1 table spoon of chia seeds blended in.

LUNCH: Steamed vegetables of choice with fresh herbs, drizzled with olive oil and crushed pumpkin seeds.

Combine this with 1/2 cup organic brown rice and a handful of almonds.

DINNER: Salad of fresh rocket leaves with thinly sliced strips of red capsicum, slices of fresh mushrooms and onions. Sprinkle with sunflower seeds. Toss with virgin olive oil, lemon and fresh herbs.

SNACKS: Drink as much water, unsweetened herbal tea as you wish during the day. Aim for at least 8 glass of water within the day. Make a trail mix of nuts and seeds like walnuts, almonds, pumpkin seeds, sunflower seeds, melon seeds, chia seeds and flax seeds. Eat low GI fruits like guava, pear, apple, orange, strawberries, peach, plums and apricots.

Start the morning with half a lemon squeezed into warm water or cleansing herb tea.

Follow with a brisk walk, bike ride, yoga or swimming

BREAKFAST: Make a fruit compote of dried prunes, apricots, peaches and apples pre-soaked in filtered water and sprinkled with flaked almonds and 2 tablespoon of ground flaxseeds. Have it with some plain yogurt.

LUNCH: Lentil and vegetable soup with 1/2 cup of brown rice and amaranth.

DINNER: Raw Papaya and Carrot Salad

SNACKS: Drink as much water, unsweetened herbal tea as you wish during the day. Aim for at least 8 glass of

water within the day. Make a trail mix of nuts and seeds like walnuts, almonds, pumpkin seeds, sunflower seeds, melon seeds, chia seeds and flax seeds. Eat low GI fruits like guava, pear, apple, orange, strawberries, peach, plums and apricots.

DAY 7

Start the morning with half a lemon squeezed into warm water or cleansing herb tea.

Follow with a brisk walk, bike ride, yoga or swimming

BREAKFAST: Coconut banana power smoothie

LUNCH: Lentil and vegetable soup with tossed greens, dressed with olive oil and a splash of lemon juice. Accompany with a handful of raw almonds and raisins.

DINNER: Grilled mushrooms with green salad, sweet potato mash and 1/2 cup of brown rice

SNACKS: Drink as much water, unsweetened herbal tea as you wish during the day. Aim for at least 8 glass of water within the day. Make a trail mix of nuts and seeds like walnuts, almonds, pumpkin seeds, sunflower seeds, melon seeds, chia seeds and flax seeds. Eat low GI fruits like guava, pear, apple, orange, strawberries, peach, plums and apricots.

Congratulations, you have finished your 7 days cleanse. You should be feeling fantastic and sparkling with vitality and your face should look fresh and rejuvenated. The best news is that you should now be motivated to continue feeding the best food to your body and look and feel healthy inside and out.

Detox diets are supposedly to help "clean out the system" but many people think they will lose weight if they try these diets. Here's the truth:

• **Detox diets are not recommended for teens.** Normal teenagers need lots of nutritional goodies — like enough calories and protein to support rapid growth and development. So diets that involve fasting and severe restriction of food are not a good idea. Some sports and physical activities require ample food, and fasting does not provide enough fuel to support them. For these reasons, detox diets can be especially risky for teenagers.

• **Detox diets aren't for people with health conditions.** They're not recommended for people with diabetes, heart disease, or other chronic medical conditions. Detox diets should be avoided if you are pregnant or have an eating disorder.

• **Detox diets can be addicting**. That's because there's a certain feeling that comes from going without food or from having an enema — for some, it's almost like the high other people get from nicotine or alcohol. This can become a dangerous addiction that leads to health problems, including serious eating disorders, heart problems, and even death.

• **Detox supplements can have side effects.** Many of the supplements used during detox diets are actually laxatives, which are designed to make people go to the bathroom more often, and that can get messy. Laxative supplements are never a good idea because they can cause dehydration, mineral imbalances, and problems with the digestive system.

- **Detox diets don't help people lose fat.** People who fast for several days may drop pounds, but most of it will be water and some of it may be muscle. Most people regain the weight they lost soon after completing the program.

- **Detox diets are for short-term purposes only.** In addition to causing other health problems, fasting for long periods can slow down a person's metabolism, making it harder to keep the weight off or to lose weight later.

Conclusion

There have been only a small number of studies on "detoxification" programs in people. While some have had positive results on weight and fat loss, insulin resistance, and blood pressure, the studies themselves have been of low quality—with study design problems, few participants, or lack of peer review (evaluation by other experts to ensure quality).

A 2015 review concluded that there was no compelling research to support the use of "detox" diets for weight management or eliminating toxins from the body. A 2017 review said that juicing and "detox" diets can cause initial weight loss because of low intake of calories but that they tend to lead to weight gain once a person resumes a normal diet. There have been no studies on long-term effects of "detoxification" programs.

Manufactured by Amazon.ca
Bolton, ON

15237180R00050